Belly Fat Diet

Shed Excess Weight
Lose Belly Fat For Health

And Vitality

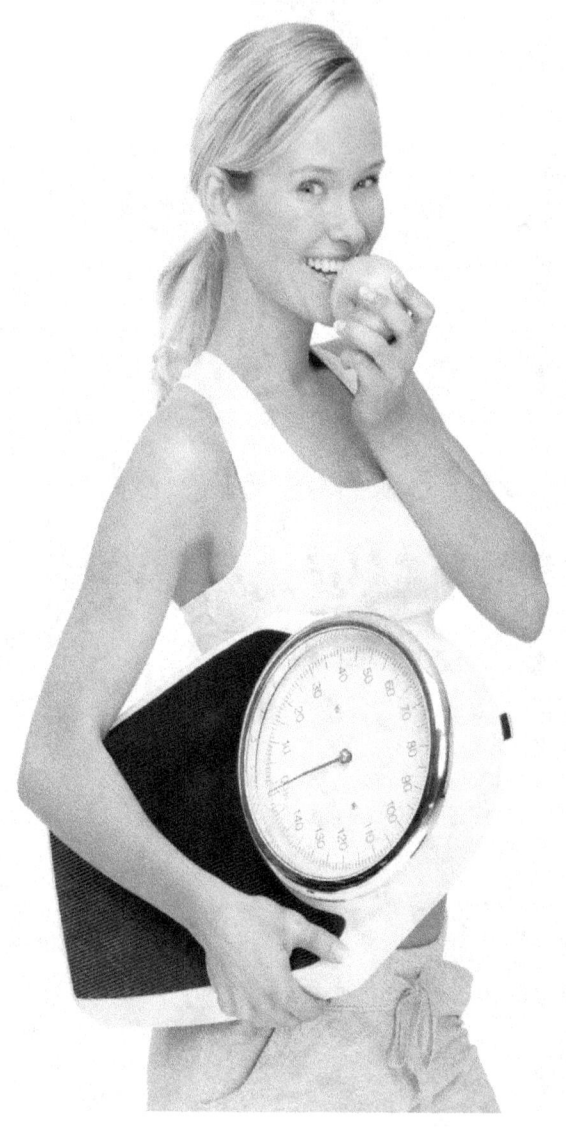

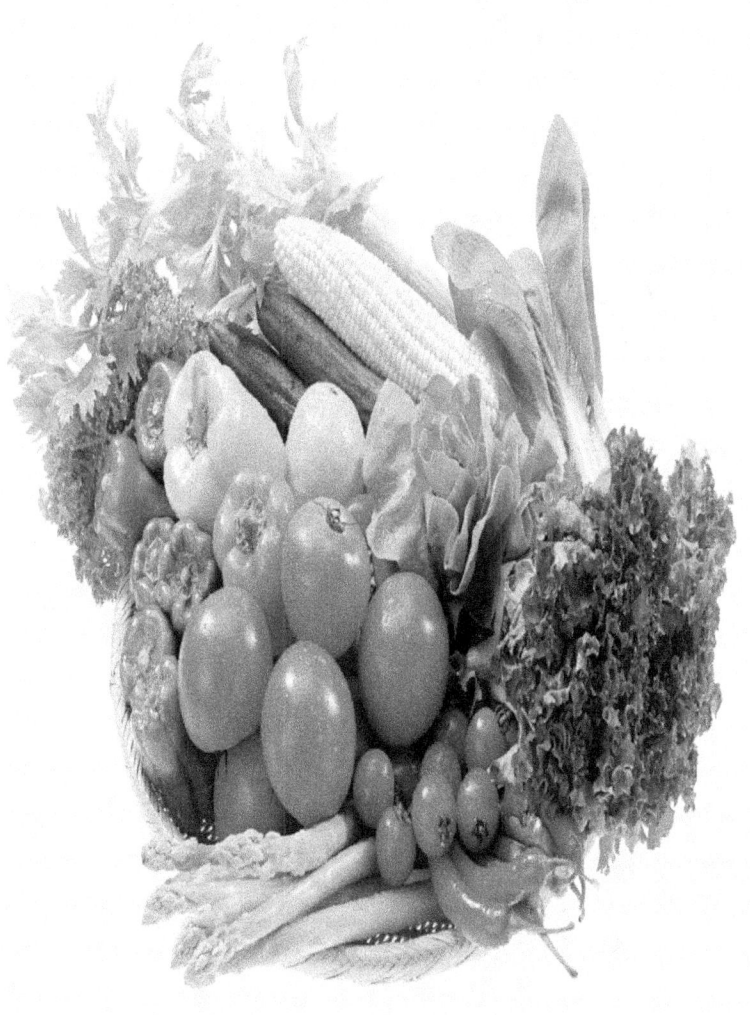

Belly Fat Diet

Shed Excess Weight Lose Belly Fat For Health And Vitality

Ashley Lopez

Copyright Notice

Disclaimer and Terms of Use

This book is a general educational health-related information product. As an express condition to reading this book, you understand and agree to the following terms. The books content is not a substitute for direct, personal, professional medical care and diagnosis.

Please see your doctor or health care provider if you are unsure of eating any of the foods in this book or participating in any of the activities as everyone has different health care needs and concerns.

The Author and/ or Publisher of this book is not responsible in any manner whatsoever for any consequential damages that result from the use of, or the inability to use this book.

First Printing, 2012

ISBN-13:978-1500270223

How This Book Will Help You

In this short book you will find proven tips and guide to help you lose weight fast without killing yourself with all these hard dieting methods.

This book is a guide to help you make small yet effective changes to your lifestyle and routine that will in time become second nature to you. The idea is that you will not be making these changes for a specific time period. You are making them into habits, so they will eventually become part of your day to day living.

You will also learn about visceral fat, how much fat is too much, belly fat fighting tips, learning the truth about the "Good Fat": Omega-3 and why you need it and much, much more.

I hope this is the dieting guide you have been looking for, packed with strategies and easy to follow.

Contents

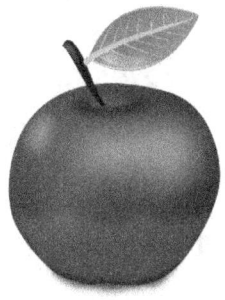

Preface: Belly Fat Syndrome

In a dream world we would all be completely without belly fat. Though, those of us who are thinner may think that they don't have to worry about it, belly fat is a problem for everyone.

In fact, some of it might even be using the area around your organs as hiding place, just waiting to cause serious health problems for you when it reaches levels which are unsafe. Whether you're a size 0 or a size 14, belly fat is present, and doesn't discriminate based upon your weight or pant size.

You might be wondering where belly fat comes from, or why it's so dangerous. There's a good chance that you've even considered how you can get rid of it, especially in times when a big party is quickly approaching or you have a wedding to attend the following weekend. The soda that you just drank or the bag of chips that you just finished eating could be to blame for your pants not zipping up quite as easily as they did before. However, bloating in the abdomen is not merely a hindrance due to the way it makes you look, but can be a source of discomfort, as well.

Don't be too discouraged though, as there is hope. Stomach bloating can be prevented by making some simple changes to your lifestyle and diet.

This isn't about stomach fat, however, but distension of the abdomen that is caused by gas. If you don't have a more serious underlying condition, such as heart disease or problems with your liver, then the only real reason for that bloating isn't water weight, but intestinal gas.

It's actually a falsehood that bloating is caused by fluid buildup in healthy adults, because the abdomen isn't the first place that fluids would gather if you're standing up; it would be present in the legs and ankles before becoming noticeable anywhere else.

What really causes the gas that makes you feel and look awful can be traced back to a variety of things, ranging from food allergies to constipation.

Before we continue on, it's important to stress that this isn't some sort of anti-fat propaganda. Your body does, after all, need a little bit of fat. Instead, this is more of a guide to understanding where this "invisible" fat is, and to figure out what different fat in different places is doing to your health, as all fat is not alike.

You see, there are essentially two types of fat: subcutaneous and visceral. We store subcutaneous fat just under the surface of our skin, such as in the abdomen and thighs. The visceral fat, however, is the more dangerous of the two, as it is stored deeper and surround the vital organs. Visceral fat, though not as noticeable, is what really poses a greater threat to us.

Introduction

Whatever They Told You about Losing Weight Is Dead Wrong...And Here's Why

Losing weight is one thing that many people have struggled with at some point in their life. For some, this fight can be on going. It can include the pleasures of getting into that pair of jeans and losing those undesirable pounds, and feeling amazing.

Only to realize that in just a few weeks the weight comes stacking back on, adding a pound or two extra with it. There are some fortunate people who have been slim all their lives and can eat whatever they want without putting any extra weight on. And then, there are some who make weight loss look effortless.

The content in this book is helpful information to assist you in making modest yet powerful changes to your lifestyle and your routine that will become second nature for you. The secret is that, you will not make these changes for a specific time period. You're making a lot into habits, so they will ultimately become part of your day-to-day living.

The primary reason lots of weight loss plans tend not to work, is due to the fact that they are viewed as a temporary fix. They can be time consuming, very rigorous, and hard to fit into your daily routine.

The content in this book supplies everything you need to create your own strategy. You can review the information and take the ideas that are the most important to you and then put them collectively in a sense that fits in with your regular lifestyle. All the advice is taken from recent research and will not put your health at risk.

The Importance of Setting Goals to Lose Weight

The one thing that all successful individuals have in common is setting goals. Whether it's for weight loss or other personal reasons; goal setting has played a Hugh part in helping them to accomplish their objectives. When looking at ways to achieve and keep a healthy weight, setting goals is always a great way to begin. Setting goals for weight loss is a very powerful method, because it allows you to feel excited and motivated about getting to where you would like to be.

However, they could also have the opposite result. Poor personal goal setting can result in frustration and disillusion, eventually causing you to give up on yourself. So getting it right from the start and to do it correctly is crucial.

Goals must be set in ways that enables one to reach them. It's important for you to measure your fitness by weighing yourself to see how much weight you've lost in a week or by how far you can run.

Having the ability to measure your progress is a valuable tool for keeping you motivated. Reaching your goals is essential as it will have a huge impact on your motivation. In order to achieve your long term goal, you'll likely need to break it down into chunks that are achievable.

Furthermore, give your goal a time frame. Time frame provides you with a structure in which to work. By setting goals such as the exact amount of pounds you would like to lose without setting a timeframe makes it easy to go off track.

Chapter 1

Understanding Visceral Fat

It's important to know that fat doesn't just simply sit there in our bodies; it secretes substances just like any other organ. While the visceral variety of fat does provide cushioning to our organs, it also puts out a substance that can then be absorbed by those surrounding organs, such as the lungs and the kidneys.

Visceral fat cells can even release chemicals that can lead to cancer, insulin resistance (diabetes), breast cancer, colon cancer, dementia, and heart disease, amongst other conditions.

Visceral Fat

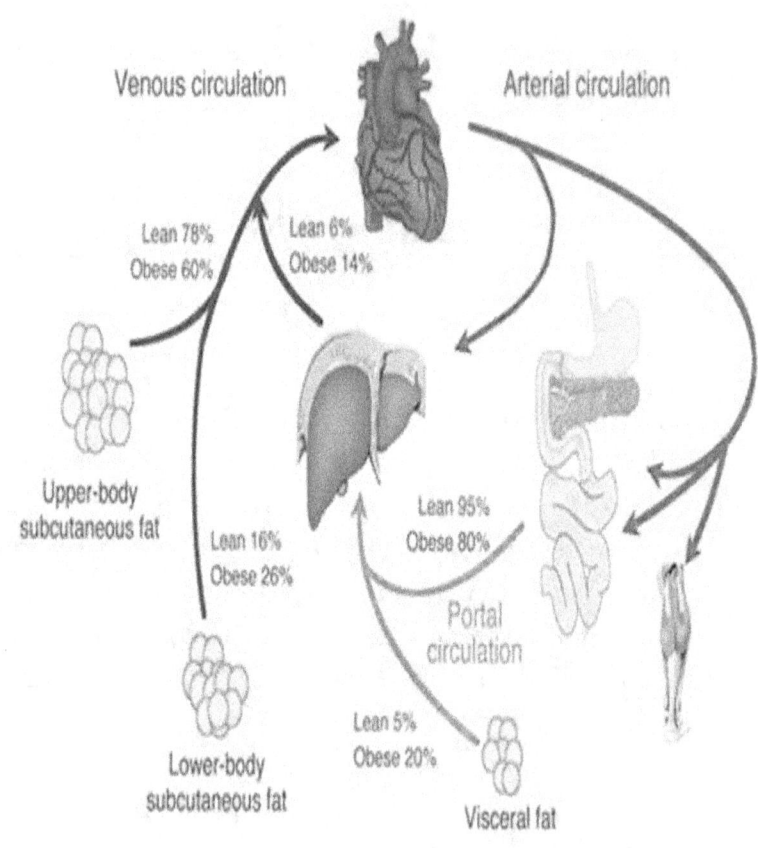

Venous circulation

Arterial circulation

Lean 78%
Obese 60%

Lean 6%
Obese 14%

Upper-body
subcutaneous fat

Lean 16%
Obese 26%

Lean 95%
Obese 80%

Portal
circulation

Lower-body
subcutaneous fat

Lean 5%
Obese 20%

Visceral fat

How Do You Get Visceral Fat?

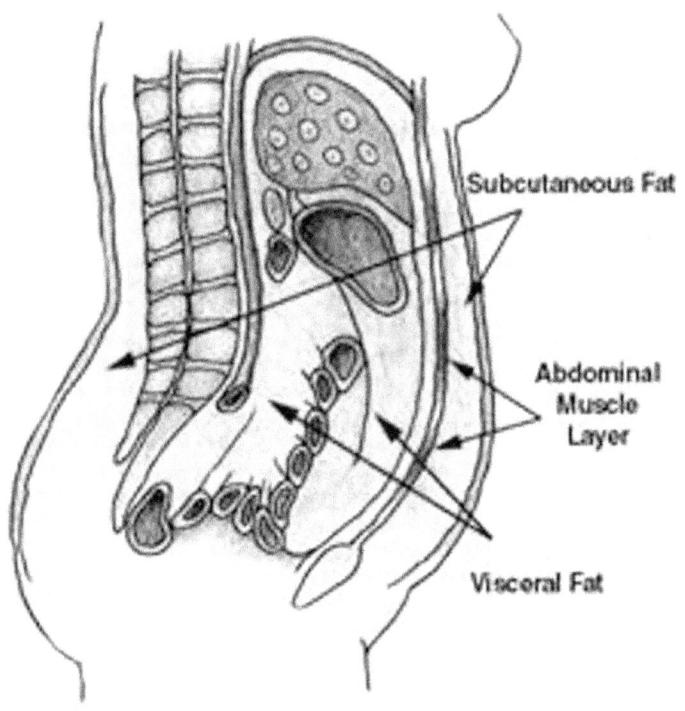

Every person on earth has visceral fat and subcutaneous fat, regardless of your weight or size. That's one thing we all have in common. However, where we differ is when it comes to where we store that fat, which all depends upon things like our genes, lifestyle choices and age, as well as gender.

For instance, men store more visceral fat than subcutaneous, while women are the exact opposite until they hit menopause. Therefore, it's inevitable that you will have some sort of fact within your body, but it becomes a concern when you've collected too much of it.

Obese people simply run out of space to store fat, so their bodies begin to store it around their vital organs instead. More and more obese people are beginning to get Fatty Liver Disease, when it was once a condition reserved for mainly alcoholics. This is due to the fact that the fat is now even retreating into the organs themselves and around the heart.

Chapter 2

How Much Fat Is Too Much?

If you would like to invest the money into seeing just where your fat is stored, then you can pay to have an MRI or CT scan performed, but there are also a number of things that you can do to figure out where you're storing your fat that are easy and free. If you're a woman and your waist circumference is greater than 35 inches, and a man who has a waist circumference of over 40 inches, then you may have dangerous levels of visceral fat.

Here are a few tips to getting an accurate waist measurement, as set forth by the National Heart Lung and Blood Institute:

- While standing up, exhale before you measure; be sure not to hold your breath.

- The tape measure should be wrapped around your middle, and should stretch across your navel.

- The bottom of your tape measure should be right above your hip bones.

You can also measure your hips, as well. Your waist-to-hip ratio will also provide you with an accurate calculation of where your fat is distributed. The Western Journal of Medicine states that above 0.8 for women and above 0.9 for men is a healthy ratio.

In order to get your hip measurements, simply place the tape measure around your hips while standing, and make sure that you measure around the part of your hip that protrudes. Divide your waist measurement by your hip measurement to get your waist-to-hip ratio.

Belly Fat

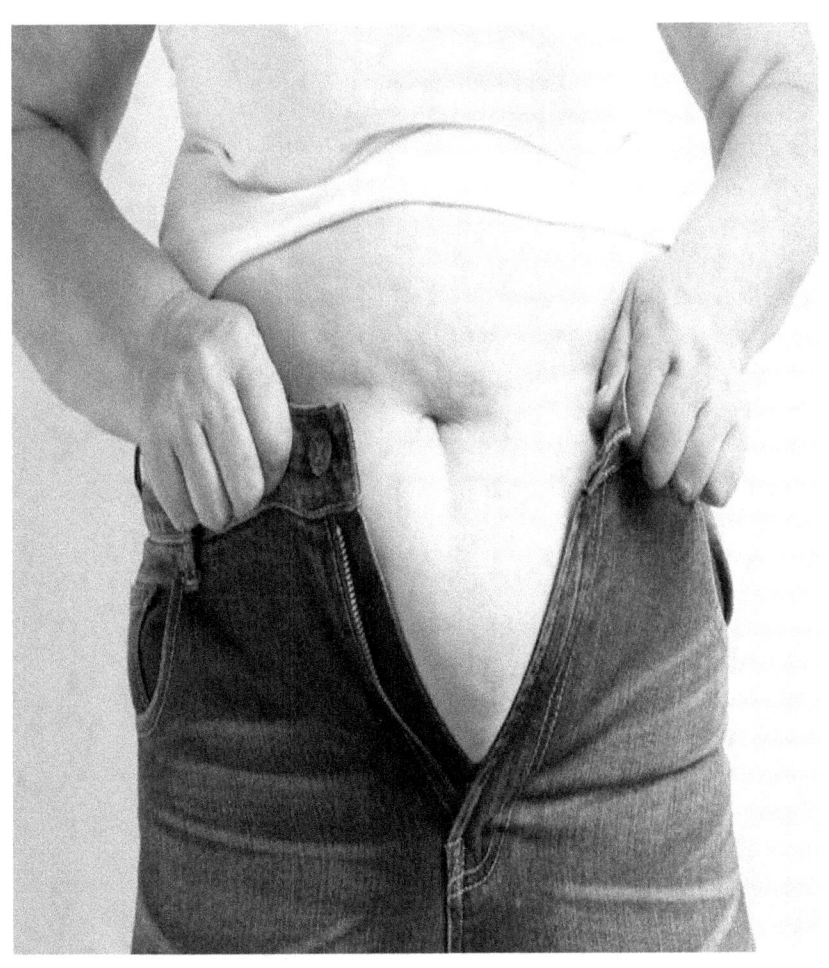

Chapter 3

It All Comes Down To Pears And Apples

You often hear the term "BMI" thrown around, which is the relation of your height to your weight, but that number doesn't really tell you where your fat is being stored, simply how much of it you have. What really matters, when it comes to your health, is your shape. Are you an apple or a pear? It's believed that having a pear shape is safer than having an apple shape.

An apple shape indicates that you probably have more abdominal fat; therefore, more than likely, you have more visceral fat. While those that are pear shaped store most of their fat, which tends to subcutaneous, in their thighs and hips.

What About Thin People?

Usually, if you're at a healthier weight, then you'll have less visceral fat. However, if your genes are set to have more visceral fat, then you will, even if you're thin. Thin people whose genetic makeup tends to store visceral fat will, just like overweight people, run a higher risk of developing certain medical conditions, such as higher cholesterol and higher blood sugar.

This is due to their insulin resistance. If you are thin, and tests have shown that these conditions are present within your body, then it may be a sign that you're storing this sort of fat. Thin people can combat this, though, by maintaining a healthy diet and exercise routine.

Pear And Apple Shape

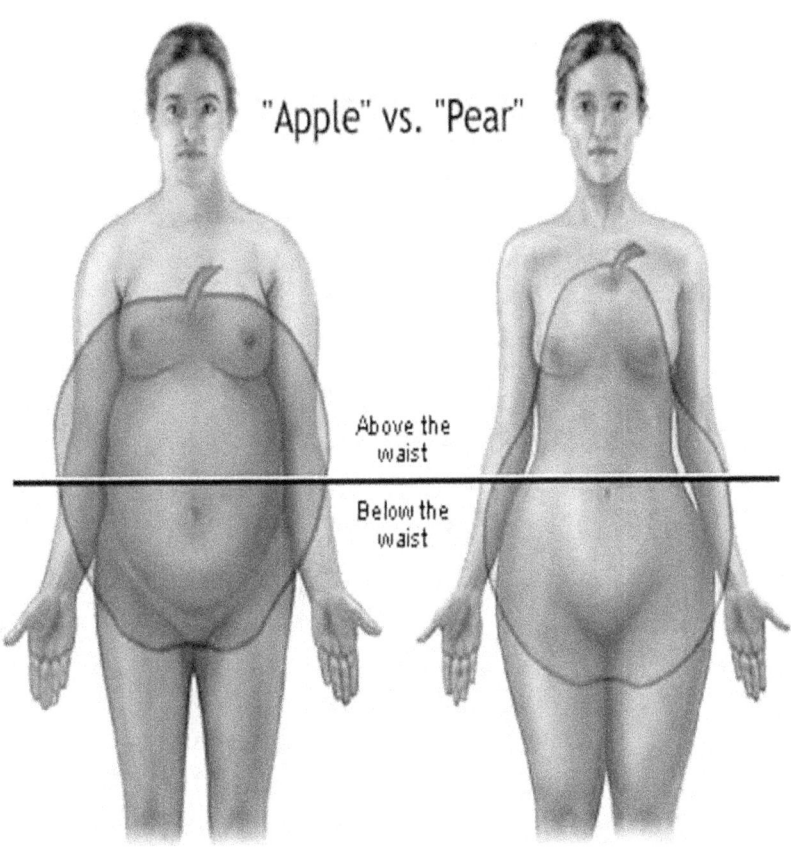

Chapter 4

What Can I Do To Finally Control And To Get Rid Of Visceral Fat?

There are, essentially, four things that you can do to control visceral fat: diet, sleep, exercise, and managing your stress levels. Here is how each can reduce the risk of accumulating visceral fat:

Diet

There isn't any diet that will get rid of only visceral fat, unfortunately. However, when you shed the pounds, it's typically your belly fat that goes first. Also, try including more fiber in your diet, as research has shown that people who eat at least 10 grams of soluble fiber each day usually retain less visceral fat. That might seem like a lot of fiber, but it's really only 2 small apples or a half a cup of pinto beans.

Rich In Fiber Beans

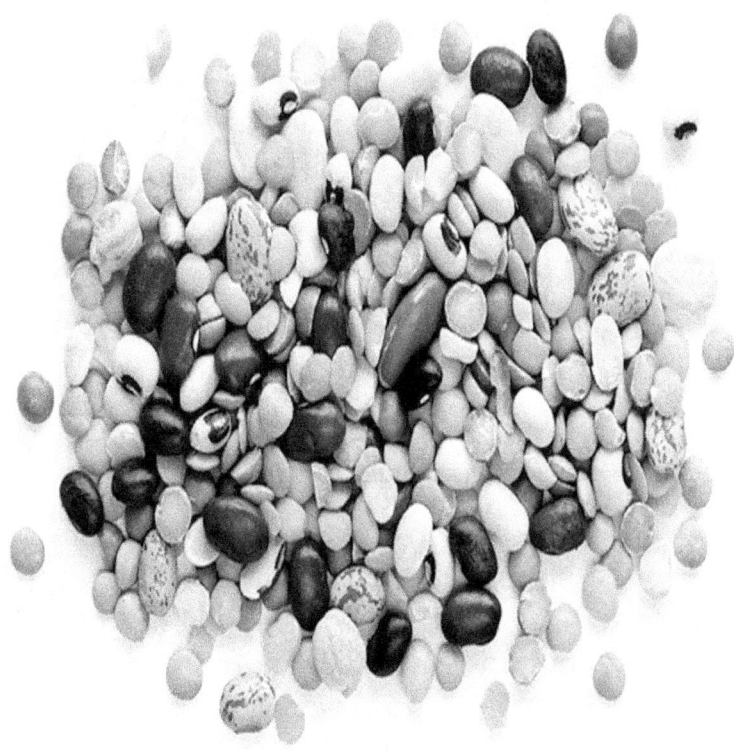

Sleep

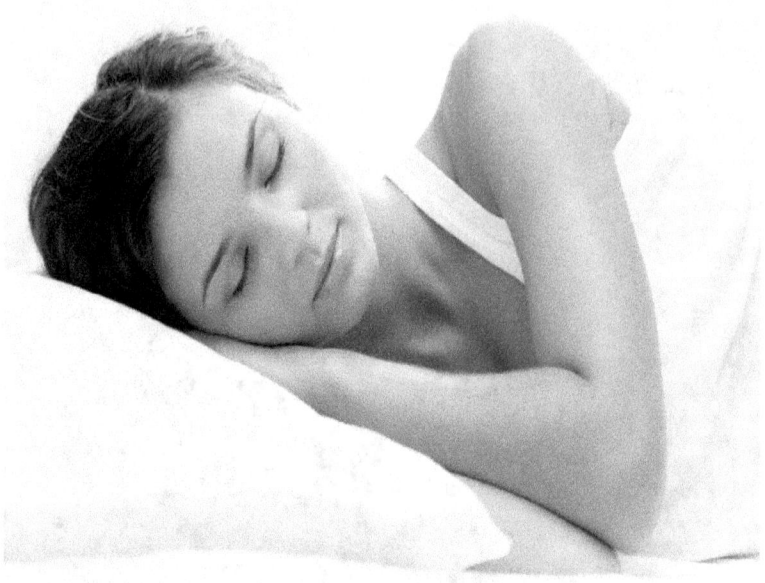

Believe it or not, too much sleep or not enough sleep can make a big difference when it comes to visceral fat. A study conducted in sleep; showed that sleep may contribute to visceral fat build up. Over a five year period, people who sleep less than 5 hours or more than 8 actually gained more visceral fat than people who slept around six or seven hours each night.

Exercise

Don't worry about trying to exercise the fat away in certain areas, as a good aerobic workout will allow for you to lose weight throughout the entirety of your body. There really aren't any certain workouts that can target key fatty spots, and studies have shown that a vigorous aerobic workout will help you to lose visceral and subcutaneous fat, as well as fat deposits in your liver.

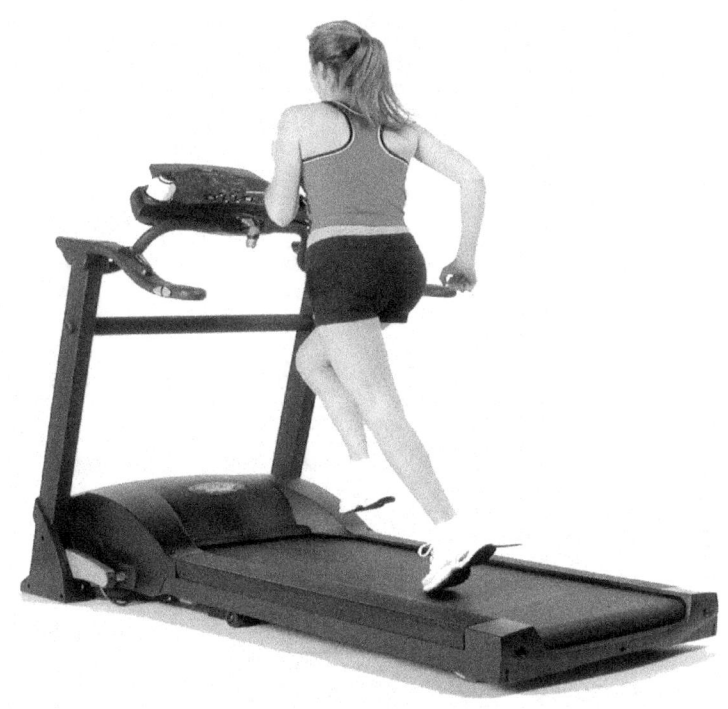

It has also been shown to slow the accumulation of visceral fat as you grow older. Try working out for 30 minutes a day, 4 times a week. You can do anything from walking to using an elliptical machine to get in some vigorous aerobic exercise. If your current physical condition won't allow for you to go all out, then just ease into your workouts and increase the difficulty of them as you go along.

On the other hand, a sedentary lifestyle will lead to a greater store of visceral fat. So, get out there and play a game with your children or join a Zumba class to raise your heart rate for around 30 minutes a day, at least 4 times a week. Ask your doctor if you're unsure if you're fit enough for physical activity, just to be safe.

Stress Management

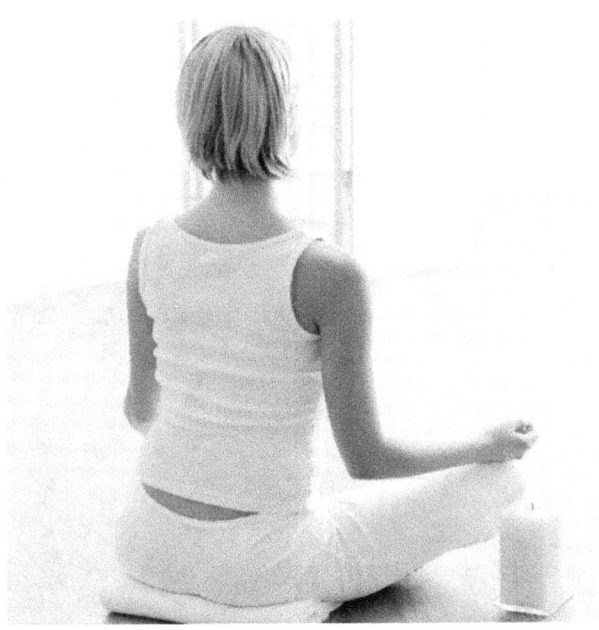

We all know how stress can impact our lives, but it might just surprise you that high levels of it can actually make you store more visceral fat. There are a variety of factors which can cause stress, ranging from personal issues to discrimination within our society.

In fact, a study that was published in the American Journal of Epidemiology found that African-American women and white women who had come up against some sort of

33

discrimination within their lives stored more visceral fat than those who hadn't ever experienced it.

The stress itself is not what causes weight gain, but your response to that stress. Therefore, it's wise to find healthier ways to handle stress, such as support groups, friends, meditating, and even exercise. The International Journal of Psychiatry in Medicine published a report that stated that women who pray or meditate have lower levels of cortisone, which is the hormone that causes stress.

Chapter 5

Belly Fat Fighting Tips

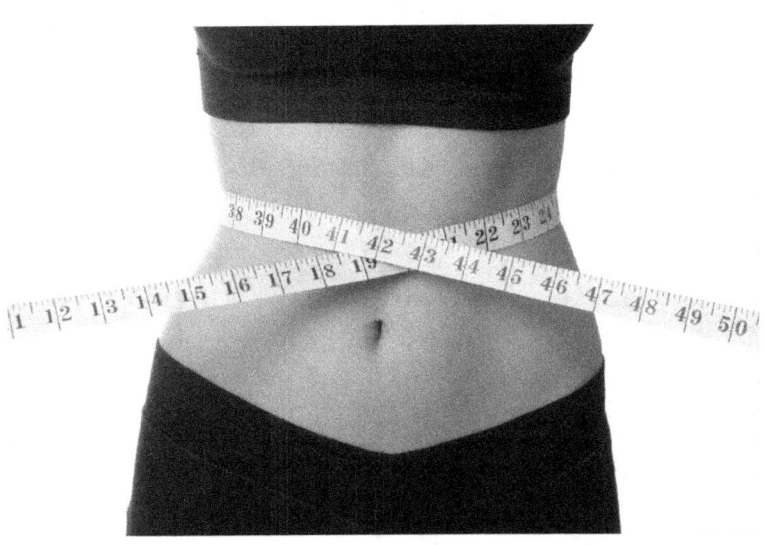

What would a guide about de-bloating be without a few flat belly tips? So, without further ado, here are 10 of them that are sure to beat the bloat:

1. Fiber = Less chance of constipation. Get plenty of fiber, fluids and fitness in order to avoid constipation, as it can make you feel bloated.

Drink 6 to 8 glasses of water per day, along with 25 grams of fiber (for women) and 38 grams of fiber (for men). Also, make sure to get your 30 minute workouts at least 4 times a week.

2. Make sure you're not allergic to wheat or lactose. If you suspect that you may have wheat allergies or are lactose intolerant, then make an appointment to see your doctor.

Many people have the tendency to believe that they might have allergies, and eliminate healthy items from their diet to avoid bloating, only to find that they are not receiving adequate nutrition. So, ask your doctor first, and slowly but surely reduce the culprits from your diet.

3. Slow down when you eat. Not only will eating more slowly leave you feeling more satisfied quicker, but it can

reduce your bloating. When you eat quickly, you swallow more air, thereby causing more gas.

So, just slow down and take around 30 minutes to enjoy each meal, remembering to chew your food thoroughly.

4. Avoid carbonated drinks. It's best to stick with flavored waters or juices, rather than fizzy beverages that can cause gas.

The carbonation within beverages, such as soda or bubbly water, can create gas which gets trapped within your stomach, making you feel bloated and uncomfortable.

5. Avoid chewing gum. Chewing gum can also lead to swallowing air, which will cause gas within your stomach.

So, try to switch to hard candy, or even eating popcorn or vegetables, if you feel the urge to chew a piece of gum.

6. Sugar-Free foods can be troublesome. You really shouldn't eat any more than 2 to 3 servings of artificially sweetened foods or beverages per day, as items that contain sugar alcohols can cause bloating.

7. Watch your sodium intake. Processed foods tend to be low in fiber and high in sodium, which can cause bloating.

So, when you're at the grocery store, start paying attention to the labels on the items you purchase. Try to find products which don't contain more than 500 mg of sodium per serving.

8. Beans and certain veggies = gas. You shouldn't avoid eating beans or vegetables, as they are a great source of protein and vitamins.

You should, however, ease them into your diet and not go overboard in your consumption of them. Vegetables that tend to cause gas are broccoli, Brussels sprouts and cauliflower, so eat them in moderation. Or, if you'd like to keep eating these items, then you might want to consider taking an anti-gas product that you can buy over the counter.

9. Eat smaller meals. Try to eat 5 to 6 smaller meals throughout the day, rather than eating 3 larger meals, as this can lead to bloating and spikes in blood sugar. Make sure that the meals

you are eating, however, are still healthy and low in calories and fat.

10.   Try all natural "beat the bloat" drinks and foods. Research has shown that foods like pineapple, peppermint, and parsley, as well as peppermint tea can help to de-bloat your body.

Yogurts also contain good bacteria, which can aid in ridding your body of gas.

Chapter 6

Learning The Truth About The "Good Fat": Omega-3

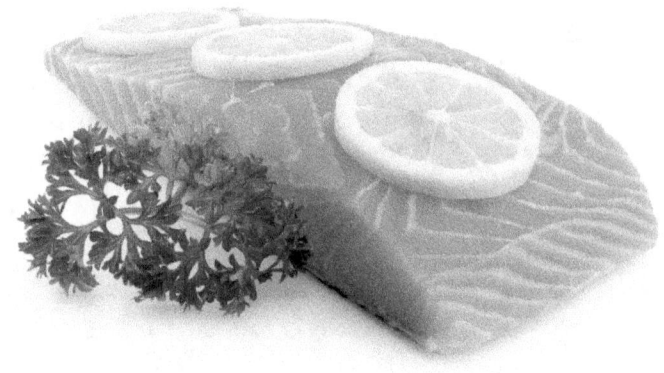

Not all fats are bad. As a matter of fact, Omega-3 fatty acids offer a variety of health benefits. They have been known to lower your risk of heart disease, and battle the symptoms of depression, cancer, arthritis, and dementia. You can find Omega-3 fatty acids in foods like salmon, leafy greens, as well as nuts. The benefits you get differ greatly from the foods that you each which contain this good fat.

The Alphabet That Makes Up the Omega-3 Family

Omega-3 fatty acids don't come in just one form. The types of Omega-3 that are found in fish, which are known as DHA and EPA, tend to offer the most health benefits. Another type of Omega-3, called AHA, is converted into EPA and DHA by the body, and is found in foods such as spinach, walnuts, and flaxseed oil.

Omega-3 Fatty Acids Help To Fight Disease

It's been suggested that Omega-3 fatty acids help to reduce inflammation throughout the body, such as in joints and blood vessels. They can also decrease the levels of unhealthy fats that are found in the bloodstream, reduce

41

the risk of an abnormal heart beat, and slow down the buildup of plaque in your blood vessels. Our bodies cannot produce Omega-3, so it's important to get them via your diet.

Omega-3 Can Benefit Your Heart Health

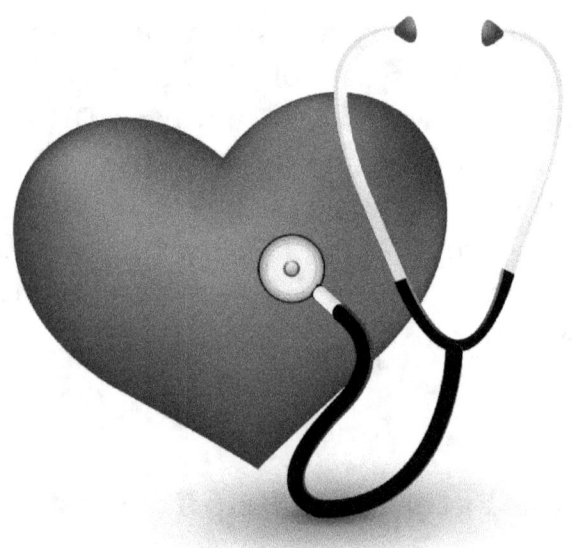

If you've suffered a heart attack before, then taking Omega-3 supplements or eating more fish can potentially lower your chances of having another. It can also lower your risk of developing an irregular heart rate or arrhythmia. Try boosting your intake of broccoli, edamame, fish, and walnuts, in order to benefit from Omega-3 fatty acids. If you have high triglycerides, then it can help you to lower those levels. However, you should consult with your doctor before increasing your intake of Omega-3, as it does contain both good and bad cholesterol, as well.

Omega-3 Can Help With Blood Pressure and Stroke

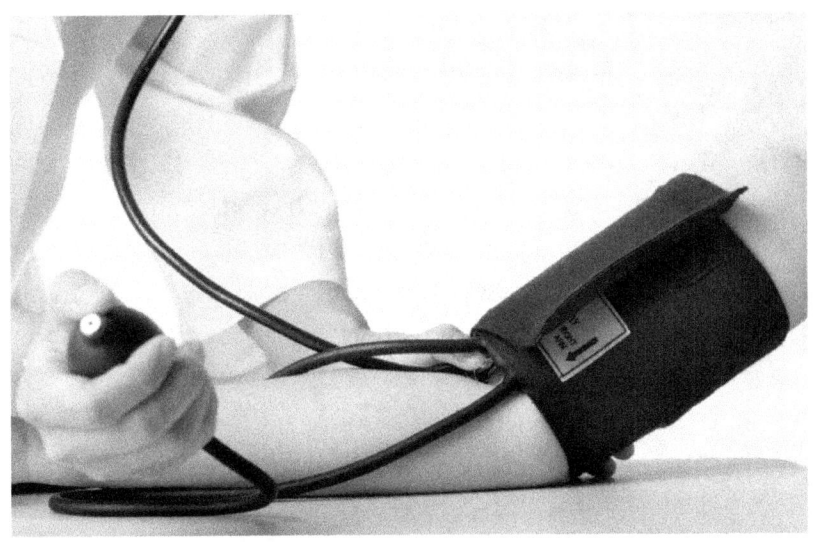

Though the impact is very small, Omega-3 fatty acids can help to lower your blood pressure. If you have high blood pressure, then changing your diet, taking your medication, and upping your fish intake (avoiding fish that is high in sodium) can help to keep your pressure at optimal levels.

Omega-3 can also help to prevent ischemic strokes, in that it prevents clotting and plaque buildup. Avoid high levels of Omega-3 though, as it has the potential to cause hemorrhagic strokes, which is the type that consists of bleeding in the brain.

Omega-3 Helps With A Variety of Medical Conditions

If you suffer from rheumatoid arthritis, then Omega-3 fatty acids can increase how well your anti-inflammatory medications work, and help to decrease the pain and stiffness in your joints. Though the findings are not concrete, it is believed that these fatty acids can also help to boost the effectiveness of antidepressants as well as your mood, for those who have been diagnosed with depression. Given that Omega-3 help with brain function and development, it's no surprise that it also helps with ADHD.

Though it's still undergoing research, it's believed that it can reduce the symptoms of attention deficit disorder. In addition, though the studies are still inconclusive, some argue that Omega-3 may improve the mental function of those who suffer from dementia, and lower the risk of being diagnosed with it.

When it comes to cancer, it's also been suggested that these fatty acids can help to reduce the risk of certain cancers, and the American Cancer Society recommends including fish in your diet, but does not suggest that Omega-3 is a cancer "cure-all".

Omega-3 Fatty Acids And The Younger Generation

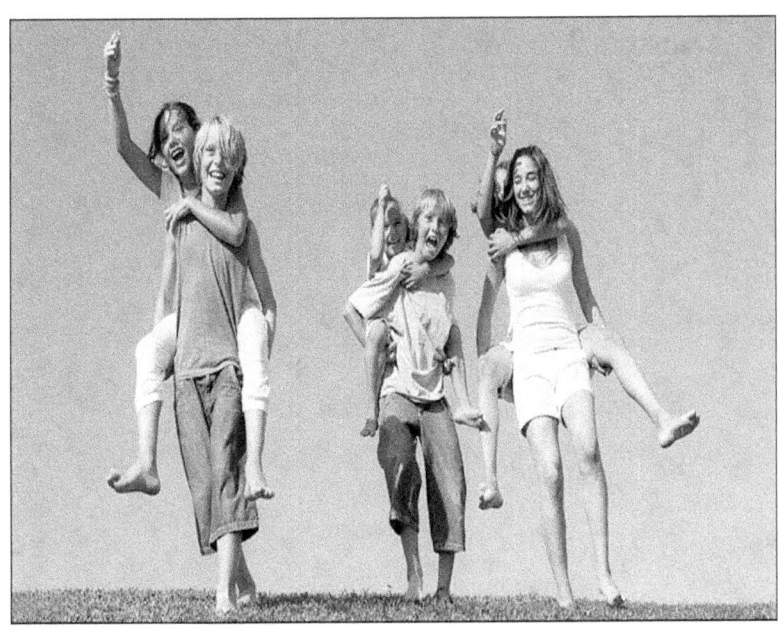

Though the American Academy of Pediatrics recommends that children do include fish in their diets, Omega-3 does not necessarily have the power to boost your child's brain power.

In fact, the Federal Trade Commission requested the supplement manufacturers stop claiming that it will do so in their advertisements and on their products. Make sure that your child's fish is not breaded or fried, and stray away from fish that are high in mercury.

Where To Find The Best Source of Omega-3

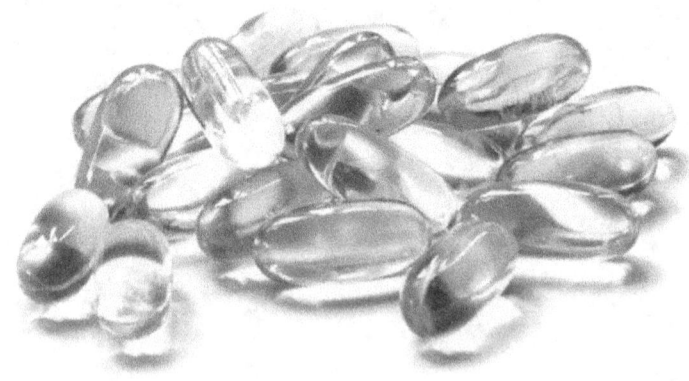

The best source of Omega-3 is fish. Some offer a higher level of it than others, such as salmon, herring, mackerel, lake trout, and anchovies. The American Heart Association suggests that you should have 2 servings of fish per week, as part of a balanced diet. Though tuna does contain Omega-3, it may also contain mercury, so it should be eaten in moderation. Albacore tuna has more Omega-3, but it has more mercury, as well.

For pregnant women, nursing women, and young children, the FDA has put forth guidelines that should be followed regarding fish consumption:

- Only eat one 6oz can of albacore tuna per week.

- Only eat fish that is lower in mercury one per week (12oz).

- Avoid eating swordfish, shark, king mackerel, and tilefish.

- Completely remove the skin and fat of the fish you eat before cooking.

Omega-3 Supplements and Vegetarian Options

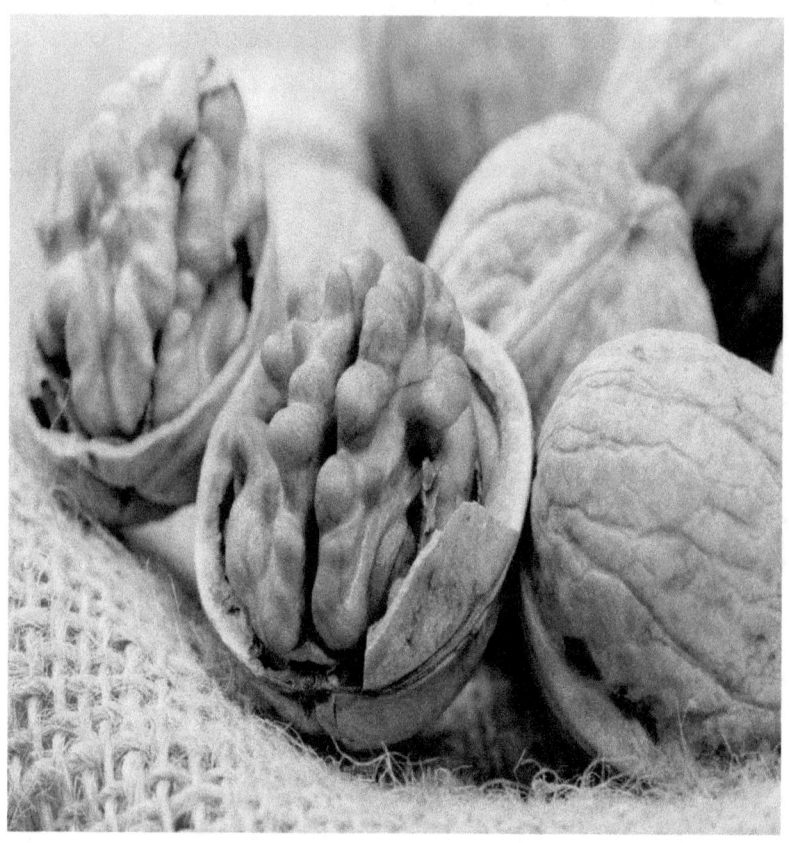

If you're not a big fish eater, then you should take 1 gram of Omega-3, if you have cardiovascular disease. High levels of Omega-3 can increase the risk of hemorrhaging, and can also diminish your Vitamin E reserves, so some supplements now include that vitamin.

48

For vegetarians, you can get your DHA fix from algae supplements. You can also eat algae that are commercially grown, or up your intake of walnuts, broccoli, flaxseed oil, and spinach.

Omega-6 Can Also Be Beneficial

Research has suggested that Omega-6, which is found in vegetable oils and nuts, may protect against heart disease. The American Heart Association recommends that you get approximately 10% of your daily caloric intake from Omega-6 fatty acids.

You should never skip meals, take laxatives or water pills, or fast in order to de-bloat. There are other options available to you that are much healthier and safer for your body. Typically, a balanced diet and exercise will help you lose that belly fat, as your abdomen is usually the first place that you'll shed those pounds when adopting a healthier lifestyle.

Also, you may want to try core strengthening exercises, such as Pilates, in order to achieve a flatter stomach and reduce belly fat. Overall, the healthiest way to look and feel better is to avoid gas-causing foods and beverages, and lead an active lifestyle.

Chapter 7

Use These Tips To Help Reach Your Weight Loss Goals!

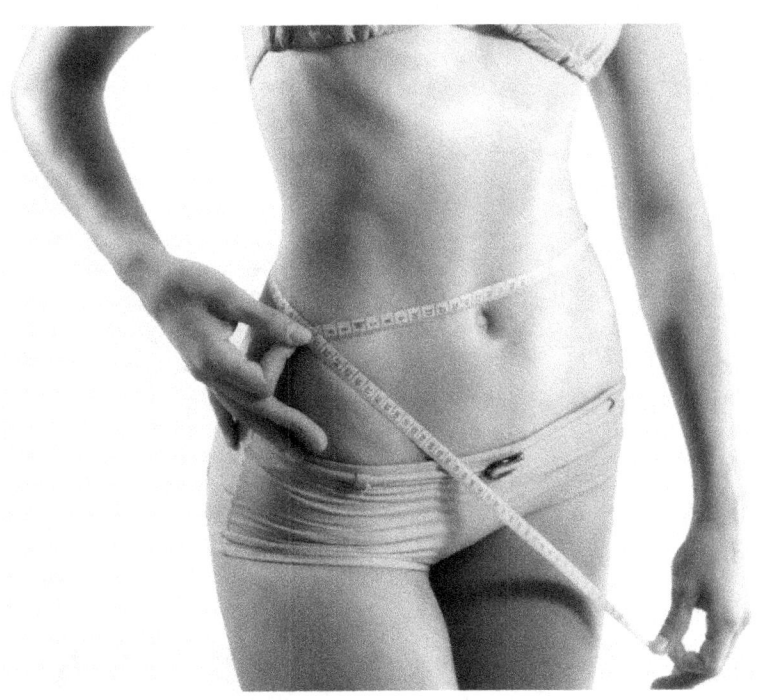

Tip No.1 Have Patience

It is important to remember to have patience when starting a weight loss plan. Pounds do not come off overnight. However, I'm going to give to you a very successful guide that will jump start the process. Remember, no matter how frustrating it may seem at times, do not give up until you reach your goal weight.

Tip No.2 Healthy Cereal

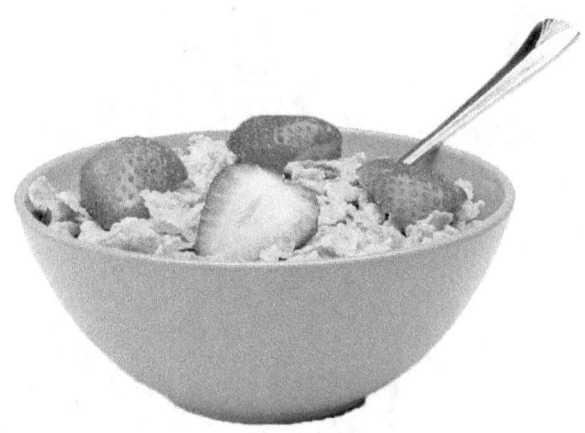

Many people enjoy having cereal for breakfast. It's quick, it's easy, and it tastes good too. Cereal is okay to have as long as you choose one that is healthy. Look for one that has at least 7 grams of fiber per serving, and is low in sugar and sodium.

Tip No.3 Eating Behaviors

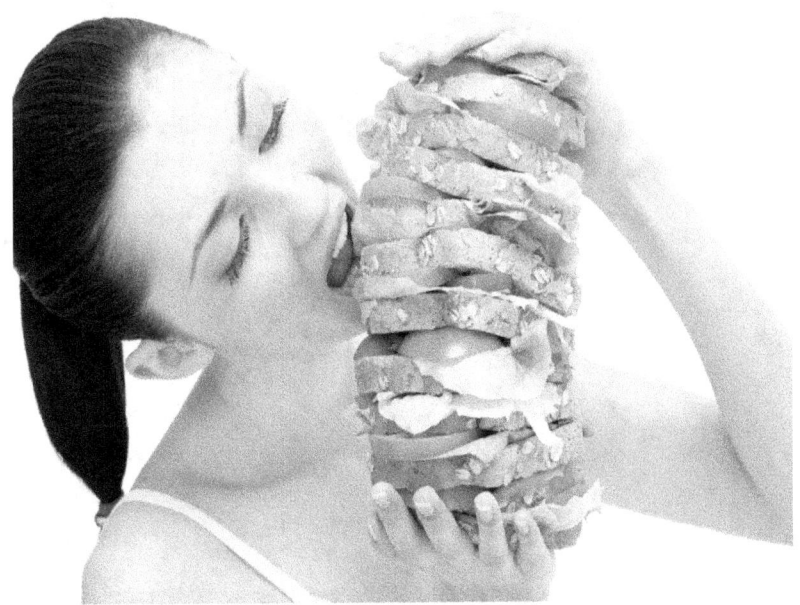

Take control of your eating behaviors to help avoid over eating. You should plan your eating so you can avoid impulse eating. When you are eating; focus on your food, not on the TV, the phone, or anything else. Don't clean your plate. You should only eat until you feel slightly full.

Tip No.4 Adding Varieties To Your Plate

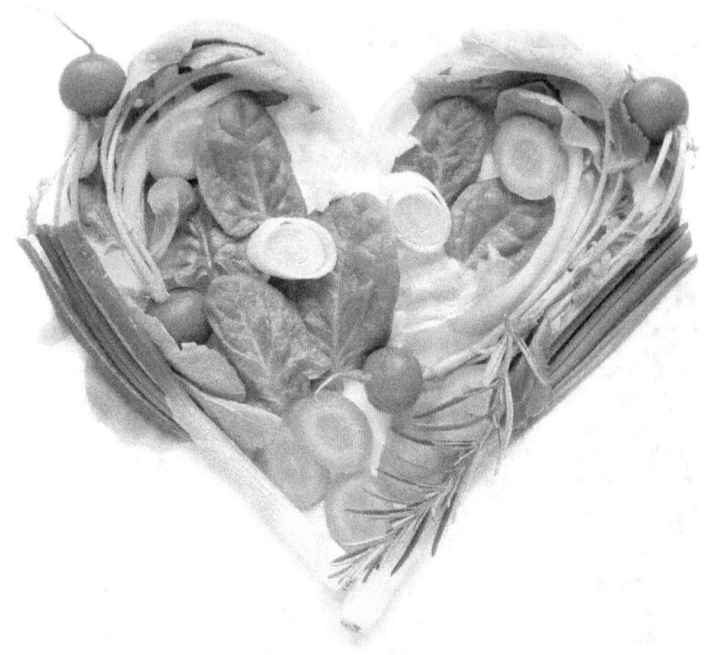

While potatoes are extremely nutritious, the monotony of brown skin and white flesh can be fairly boring. Adding other vegetables to a puree such as; cauliflower to mashed potatoes, can help boost the nutritional value. Adding colored varieties, like naturally purple or yellow varieties, can add spark and interest to a plate as well.

Tip No.5 Drinking Green Tea

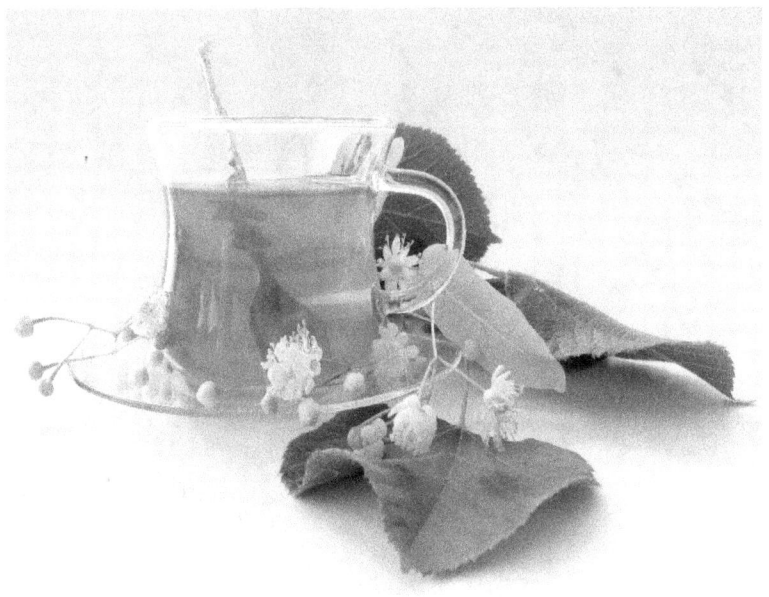

You can burn calories much faster if you boost your metabolism. This means you have to exercise, but certain foods can also help. Try drinking some green tea in the morning, or eating some chili peppers with your meals. This should give you a lot of energy and help you get rid of calories.

Tip No.6 Nutritional Boost

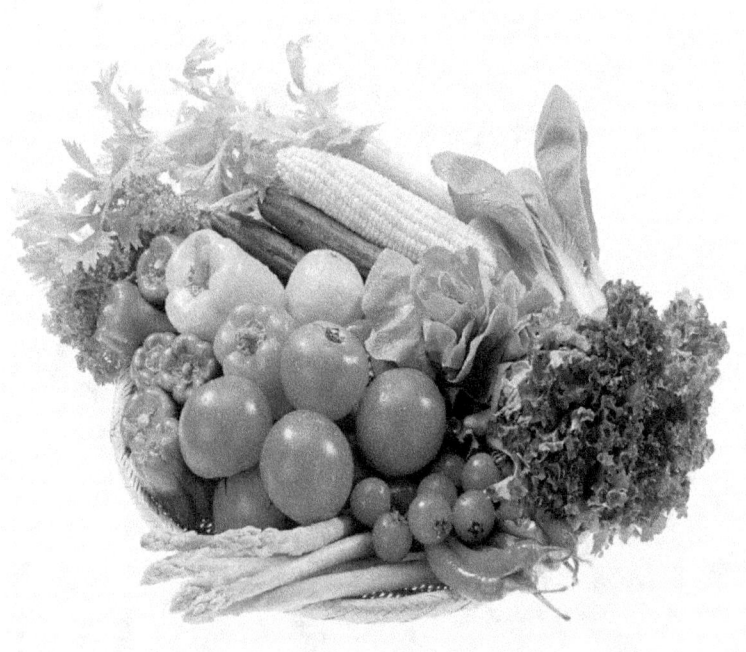

You can give any meal a nutritional boost by adding more vegetables to it. If you are eating a sandwich, go ahead and put on some tomatoes, lettuce and other vegetables that would complement it. You can add many different types of frozen vegetables to most casseroles without changing the flavor.

Tip No.7 Vegetarian Foods

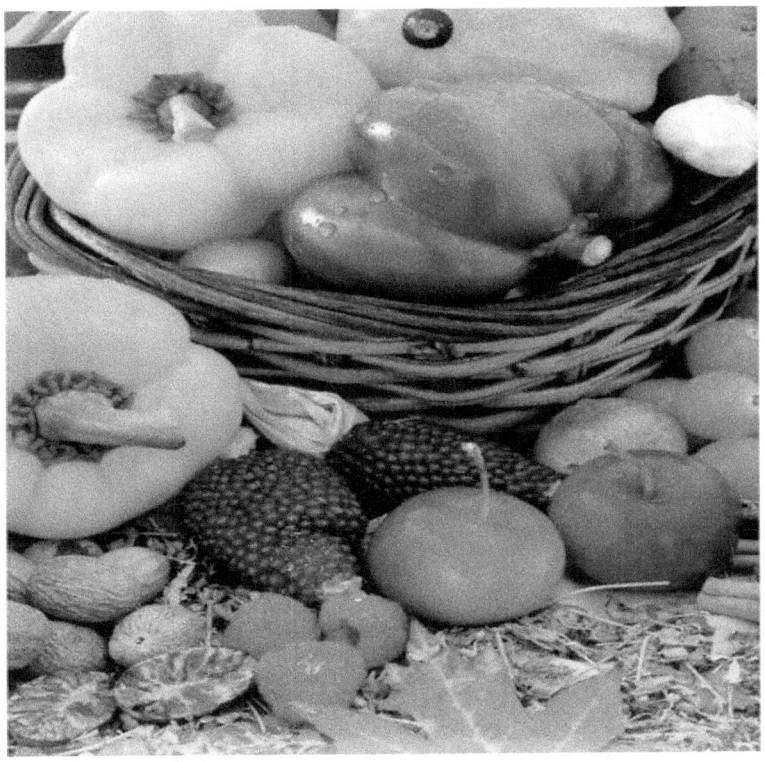

Don't think that eating vegetarian will automatically be the best choice for your health. There are many vegetarian foods available that are just as bad, if not worse than a balanced omnivorous diet. If you are going to eat vegetarian, keep it to fresh fruits, fresh vegetables, seeds, and nuts.

Tip No.8 Be Consistent

A good nutritional tip is to be consistent with the timing of when you serve your family meals. Ideally, you'll want to serve them meals around the same time every day. It's also a good idea to limit fruit drinks and soda to only meals because you can easily fill up on them.

Tip No.9 Pound Your Meat

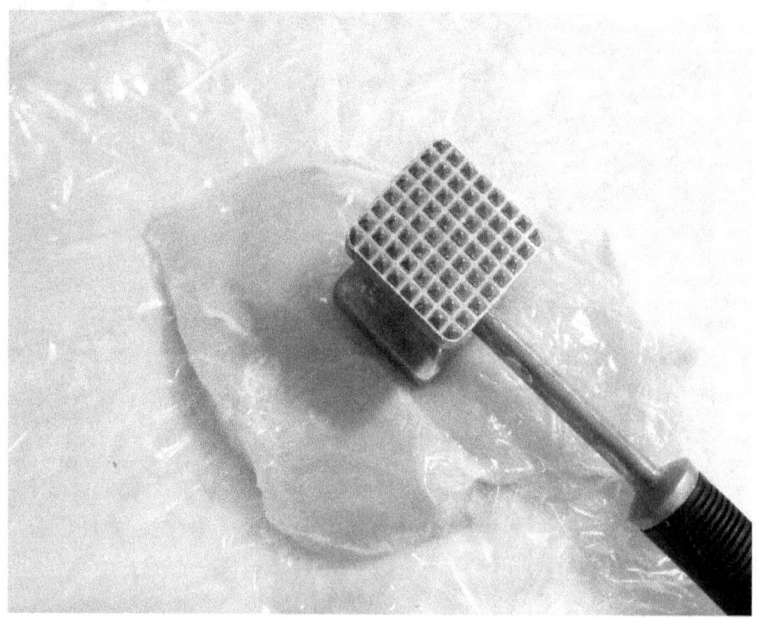

Pound your meat before you cook it. Pounding meat is not just a great way to tenderize it. Pounding it will also make your portions look larger than they actually are. This can make you feel as if you are eating more. It also serves as a great way to relieve stress.

Tip No.10 Healthy Eating Tips That Work For Busy People

A great way to prepare nourishing meals and snacks quickly "if you have a busy lifestyle" is to buy foods that are ready to consume upon opening or with little preparation. There is really no excuse not to eat healthy foods when there are plenty of options for quick eating. Some examples are low-fat deli meats, whole grain breads, frozen vegetables and fresh bagged salads to name a few.

Tip No.11 Weight Loss Program

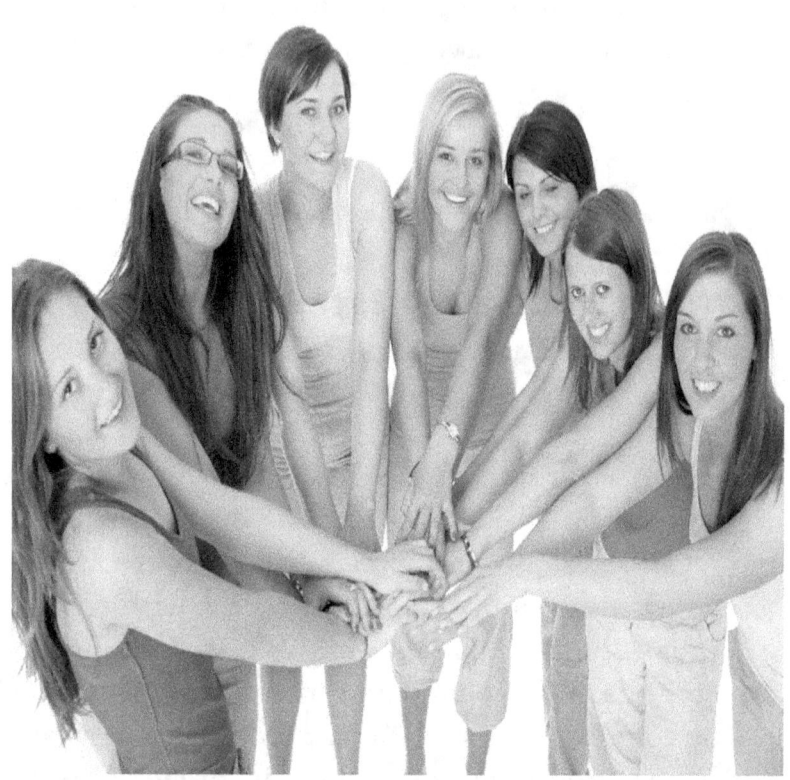

Join a weight loss program, such as Weight Watchers. Groups such as these require you to weigh in regularly, and many people find this motivating. They work harder to exercise and regulate caloric intake so that when they are weighed, everyone will see that they have lost weight. Many people find this method to be successful.

Tip No.12 Start Your Day Off With Easy To Digest Foods

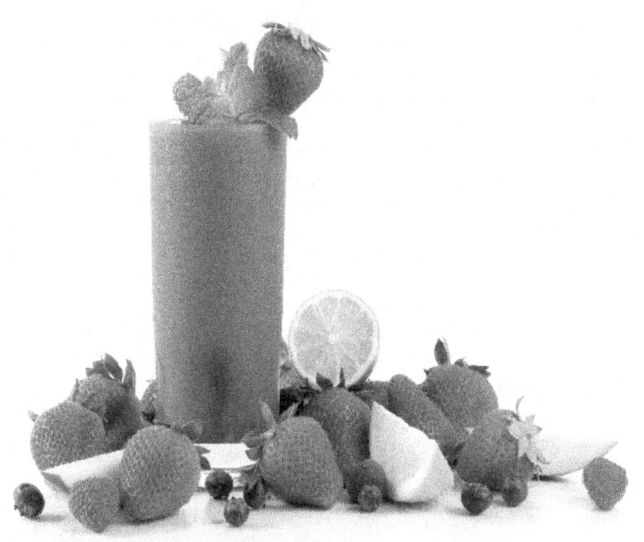

Start your day off with easy to digest foods. While many people would blanch at the sight of salad for breakfast, adding some healthy, dark, leafy greens to a smoothie can make all the difference. If you use plenty of fruits, such as strawberries or bananas, you probably will not even be able to taste the addition.

Tip No. 13 Calories Daily Intake

If you go out to eat at a restaurant, ask the waiter not to bring out bread or chips before your meal. Munching on these snacks before your main course can add a significant number of calories to your daily intake. Instead, sip a low calorie beverage and enjoy good conversation while you wait for your meal.

Tip No. 14 Taken Vitamins

If you don't like taking vitamins, ask your doctor or pharmacist about getting liquid vitamin drops. These can be added to any beverage and are especially tasty with fruit juice. The juice essentially hides the flavor and your taste buds won't even know you've taken a vitamin.

Tip No.14 Why You Should Be Eating Slowly

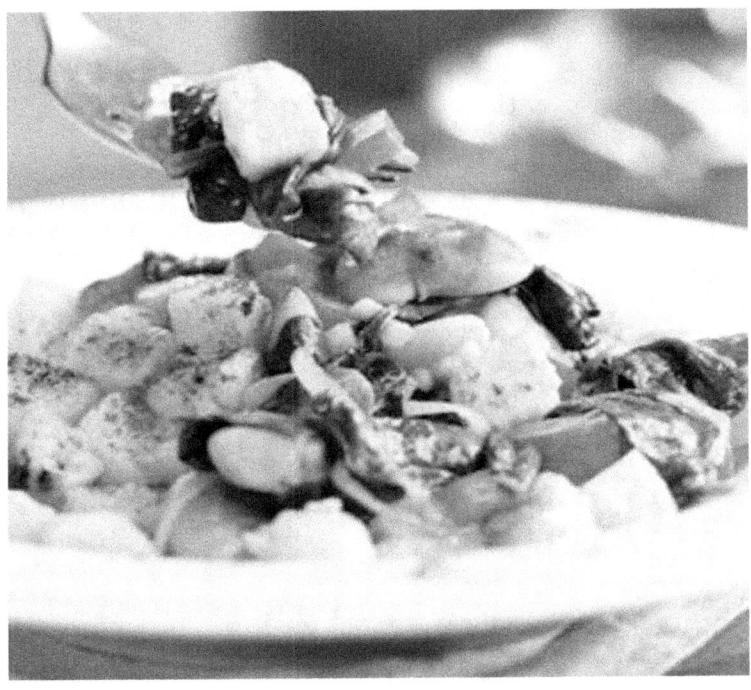

Eating slowly can help you to achieve your weight-loss goal. Did you ever notice that thin people take an awfully long time to eat their food? Eating slowly is one method that can help take off pounds. That's because from the time you begin eating it takes the brain 20 minutes to start signaling feelings of fullness.

Weight Loss Dietary Tips That Can Help You Lose Weight Faster

You should eat breakfast every day so your body has the energy it needs to function. When you wake up your body is low on energy due to not eating for 7 or more hours. Studies have shown that people feel better and eat less during the day if they start the morning with a good breakfast.

Avoid eating highly processed foods. Fuel your body with a breakfast that includes protein and carbohydrates to help you feel satisfied. Eating breakfast also keeps you from being so hungry that you end up overeating at lunch time.

When you are eating out at a restaurant, don't automatically consider the serving on your plate to be "one serving". Most restaurants serve food that is two or three times the amount dietary guidelines recommend. Take half of your plate and instantly put it in a "to go" box so that you don't end up consuming more calories than you want to.

One important weight loss tip to consider is to begin cooking your own meals as often as possible. Considering that most restaurants prepare food packed with sugar, sodium and carbs, eating out can be a serious pitfall to your diet. If you are preparing your own food, you can control what goes into it and what stays out.

Legumes and beans are also excellent sources of protein. They lack the high fat content of red meat and provide many of the essential amino acids that meat does. However, beans alone will not provide the same amino acids that meat provides, so it's necessary for a vegetarian's diet to be composed of many other sources of proteins as well. Beans are also cheap and easy to prepare.

Some people find that once they lower their carbohydrate intake, they start to lose weight. The more carbs you eat, the more carbs your body needs, and the more weight you put on.

Many dieticians recommend replacing red meats in your diet with fish. If you had tried fish once or twice in the past but really don't see it as something that you could ever eat on a daily basis, remember that there are dozens of different types of fish. Whether you opt for mackerel, mullet, snapper, sardines, or flounder, each kind has its own distinctive flavor and texture. Just because you did not like one or two kinds does not mean you will not like any of them.

Chapter 8

Nutrition Tips To Improve Your Life

There are many people that cope with stress and depression with food. If you are one of those people, go to your doctor and find a good medication that will treat depression and help control the feeling of stress. This will help you to avoid eating to cope and eliminate unnecessary calories and fat intake.

A great nutritional tip is to make sure you eat before and after your workouts. It's important to eat before you work out because your body will need plenty of fuel. It's also very important to eat within a half hour of lifting weights because it will help your muscles recover.

A lot of dieters will turn to procedures like liposuction in order to "lose" weight. Well, this isn't actually losing anything in the grand scheme of things. Yes, fat sucked out of you may cause you to appear thinner, but unless you're dealing with how you eat and exercise, you'll just put that fat back on again.

Since it is not a good idea to have so much salt in your diet you should try to find other ways to put flavor into your food. Adding fresh herbs and seasoning blends that do not contain salt are the best ways to add flavors without having to worry about salt intake.

Try to keep an upbeat attitude about your weight loss attempts. If you are able to think positively about eating in a healthy manner and convince yourself that you enjoy your workouts you will be able to think of them without dread. This will help you to stay motivated on those hard days.

Consider eating many smaller meals during the day instead of three bigger meals. Five or six small meals daily has been shown to help digestion and increase the nutritional value of the foods you eat (you absorb more nutrients). Plus, studies have shown that eating smaller meals may actually help you lose weight compared to eating three bigger meals!

Start with lessening your portion or amount, moving forward to rearranging your diet. Just omitting one snack, one extra spoonful, or one extra piece of meat to start your weight loss venture could be a great start that is motivating and not overwhelming on your appetite and regular diet.

Cook your own meals. By preparing your own meals at home instead of eating out, you can more easily control the calories contained in your meal. You are able to make healthy ingredient swaps and keep tabs on how much fat and salt are added to the dishes.

A good way to motivate you to get into shape is to have a buddy who has the same goals as you. Having a close friend or family member that wants to get into shape can help motivate you to not slack off on your goals. You can motivate each other and you can have someone to talk to about what may or may not be working out for you in your fitness efforts.

Use low-fat yogurt as a healthy alternative to chip dip. Chip dips are notoriously high in fat and calories. Low fat yogurt makes a great healthy substitute. It is thick enough to cover the chips and it packs a punch in terms of taste. Use it just like you would any other dip.

Consider joining a local sports club or class if you're having problems with losing weight. Zumba classes are very popular right now, and you shouldn't have a hard time convincing a friend or family member to join you. This makes working out fun and will make you more likely to turn exercising into a habit!

To replace the junky snacks you might have previously brought into the house, stock up on a variety of easy-to-eat fruits that you can grab when dinner is an hour away and you or your family are hungry. Great examples would be berries, grapes, apples cut into chunks and kept in acidulated water, and small or baby bananas. By keeping the fruit in clear containers in the fridge, or on the counter, will increase its "curb appeal."

Fitness Made Simple And Other Tips And Tricks For You

Being Fat Isn't Your Fault; Staying Fat Is

Physical fitness isn't just for body builders or people who have countless hours to spend at the gym. Fitness is a state of having your body at an optimum level of health. You can do this without killing yourself at the gym or eating next to nothing.

Be sure that you are getting enough protein in your diet. Protein is crucial to the development of your body and the growth of your cells. It is the energy source that keeps you going throughout the day. Protein is available from both animal and plant sources, so it is not difficult to incorporate enough protein in your meals.

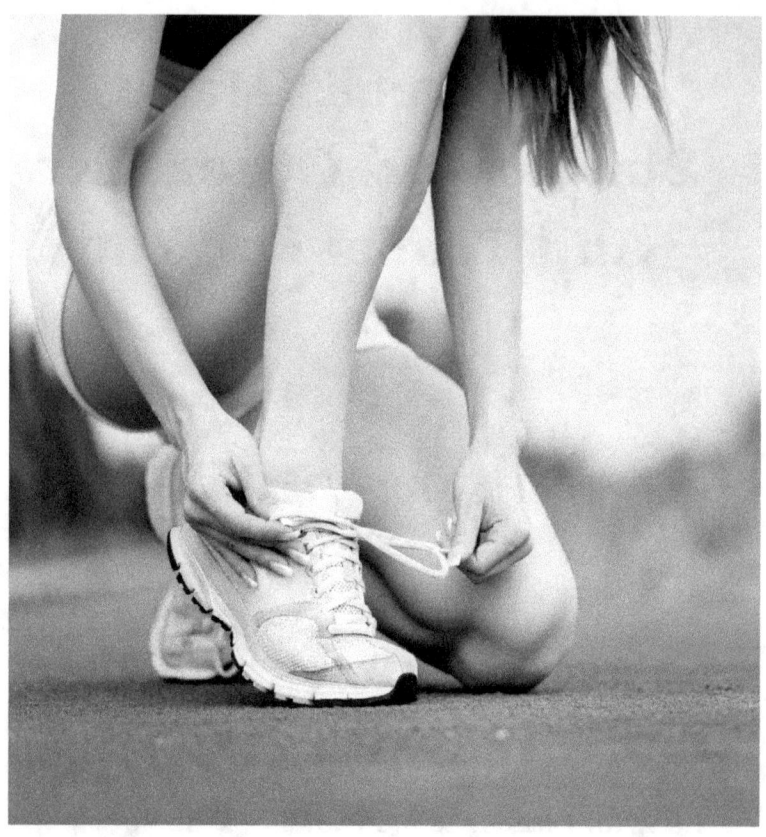

If you are using weights to do curls, bend your wrist backwards slightly. This creates a bit of tension in your forearms and biceps, forcing them to do a little extra work, which results in a better workout. It also helps to slightly increase your wrist's range of motion with each set.

When exercising, remember to keep breathing! This may seem like common sense, but during certain strength training exercise, you may find yourself holding your breath. Holding your breath can hurt your muscles. Once you've learned an exercise, focus on your breathing and try to inhale when you relax and exhale when you tighten your muscles.

When going to the gym or working out, you should have the mentality to get better and increase the amount of sets and repetitions than the previous day. This will lead to you being stronger and you will also have much more endurance than when you had first started.

Try your best to change the way you eat and drink food, choose healthier methods to get your body into shape. You want to stay away from additives such as high fructose corn syrup, which can be found in a lot of sodas. Your best bet would be to drink water and stay away from sodas and fattening drinks in general.

Chapter 9

How To Get To Your Goal Weight And Stay There

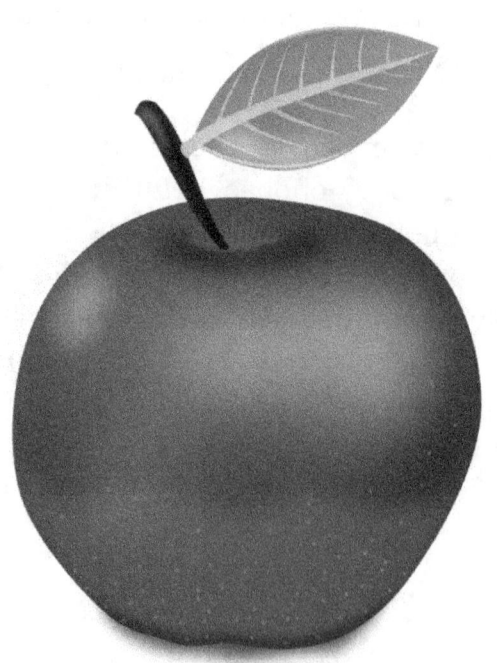

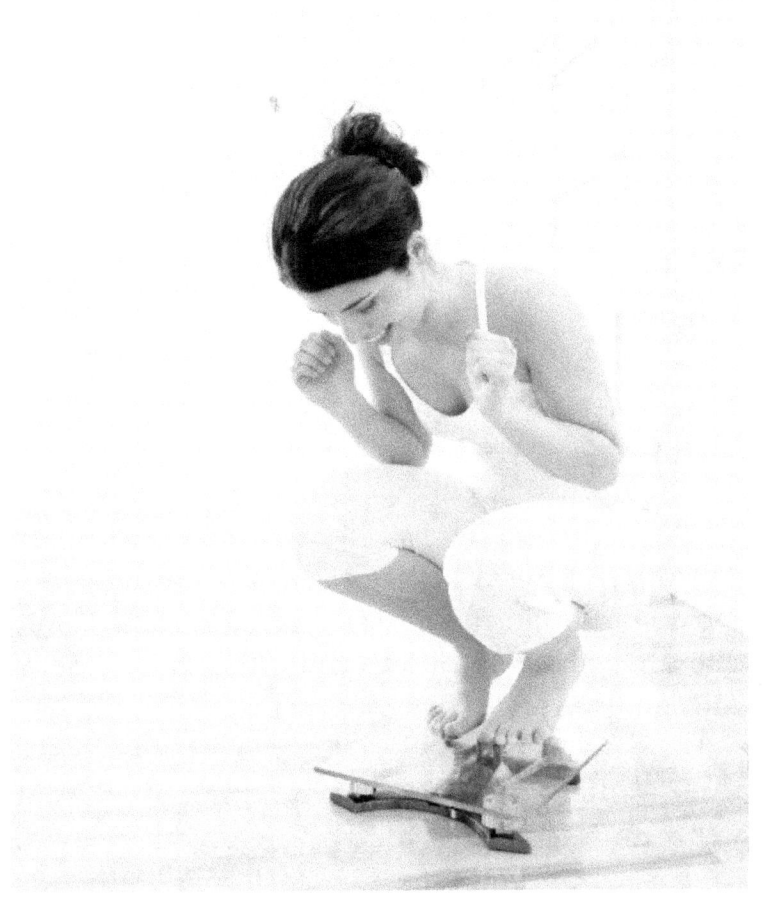

Anyone who has reached a plateau in their fitness results should try changing their workouts to incorporate different types of training. Adding resistance work or interval sets can be great ways to kick start your fitness routine. In this way, you will be able to get over the hump and begin making progress once more.

If you want to grow bigger muscles, then follow these instructions. First, you must determine how much weight to lift for a single exercise. Multiply this by how many times you lift this weight. You should aim to increase this multiplied number after every workout by lifting more weight or by increasing your volume.

If you are sick, take the time to heal instead of exercising. This is especially true if you are experiencing symptoms below the head. Your body will mostly be putting its resources towards healing itself rather than trying to build the muscle you are training for, so any work you do will more than likely be of little benefit. It's better to rest up.

After a particularly strenuous workout of a muscle group, you can help your body to recover from the stress by performing a lightly targeted workout of the affected muscles one day after. By gently engaging the muscle, you are helping it to repair itself faster by enabling your body to more efficiently deliver nutrients and blood to the area.

Although small setbacks can often feel very sad, try not to be frustrated by these experiences. You do not lose weight in one day so just one bad day will not break your diet. You can actually learn a lot from these moments and they can be overall successes in your life.

Whenever you do exercises for your abs like reverse crunches or hanging leg raises, you should round your back and roll your hips and pelvis towards your chest to better target your abdominal muscles. This will allow you to work your muscles harder and get better results more quickly.

One of the things that prevent us from having a physically fit body, are our excuses. Most people tend to say that they are too busy to find time to exercise. A good way to eliminate this is to schedule a time to work out and then stick to it until it becomes a habit.

A great way to get fit is to start eating more vegetables. Vegetables are packed with essential vitamins and nutrients and if you aren't eating enough, you aren't doing your body any favors. An easy way to make sure you're eating enough vegetables is to just toss a handful of them into a salad.

You can improve your balance by using a sofa cushion. Stand on one leg on a sofa cushion and move a medicine ball or any other heavy object from one hand to the other. Try wrapping the ball around your head and back or try each movement with your eyes closed.

Fuel your body. Always remember to eat breakfast, "this is mention a lot in this book" because it really is the best meal of the day. Before you try any form of exercise or workout, you need fuel in the form of healthy food. This will get your metabolism going, and will prevent dizziness and dehydration while exercising. Try to eat a mix of whole grains, fruit and a little dairy to get your body going in the morning.

When making a fitness plan, make sure to get expert advice rather than just doing some exercises you made up. Look around for a workout program that works for you and stick to it. The advantage of a professional program is that you're sure to work out all of your muscle groups evenly.

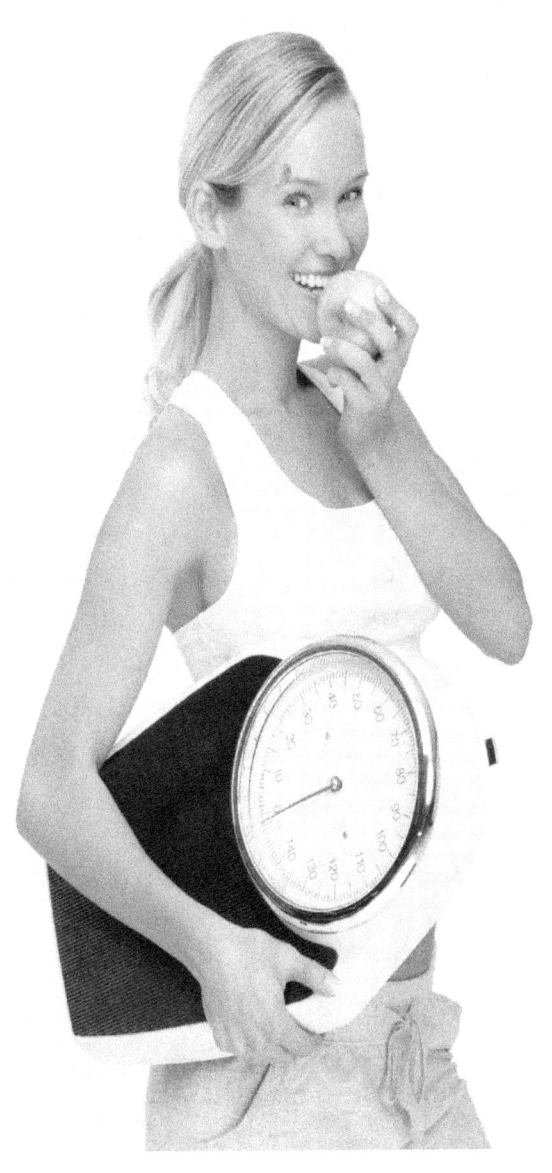

Conclusion

Don't Ever, Ever, Ever Give Up! You Must Keep Moving Forward Because There Is No Going Back. You can be fit if you want to. There is no reason for you to have to spend all of your time trying to do it. Simple changes to your daily life can make all the difference in the world. This book has shown you lots of ways that you can start to get more fit right away.

In conclusion, patience is a virtue when it comes to losing weight. As the saying goes, good things happen to those who wait. By using your patience and the information provided to you in this book, you will gradually see that losing weight and belly fat is a possibility after all. Never give up!

About The Author

Ashley Lopez is a mother 3 kids and has an active family lifestyle. Her purpose is to help men and women lose weight and obtain a healthy and balanced lifestyle without the need of depriving yourself of food or simply making weight loss and gaining better health and wellbeing feels like a monotonous or painful laborious task.

Ashley have been helping men and women within her weight loss group to possess a much more gratifying as well as healthy and fit way of living for more than six years.

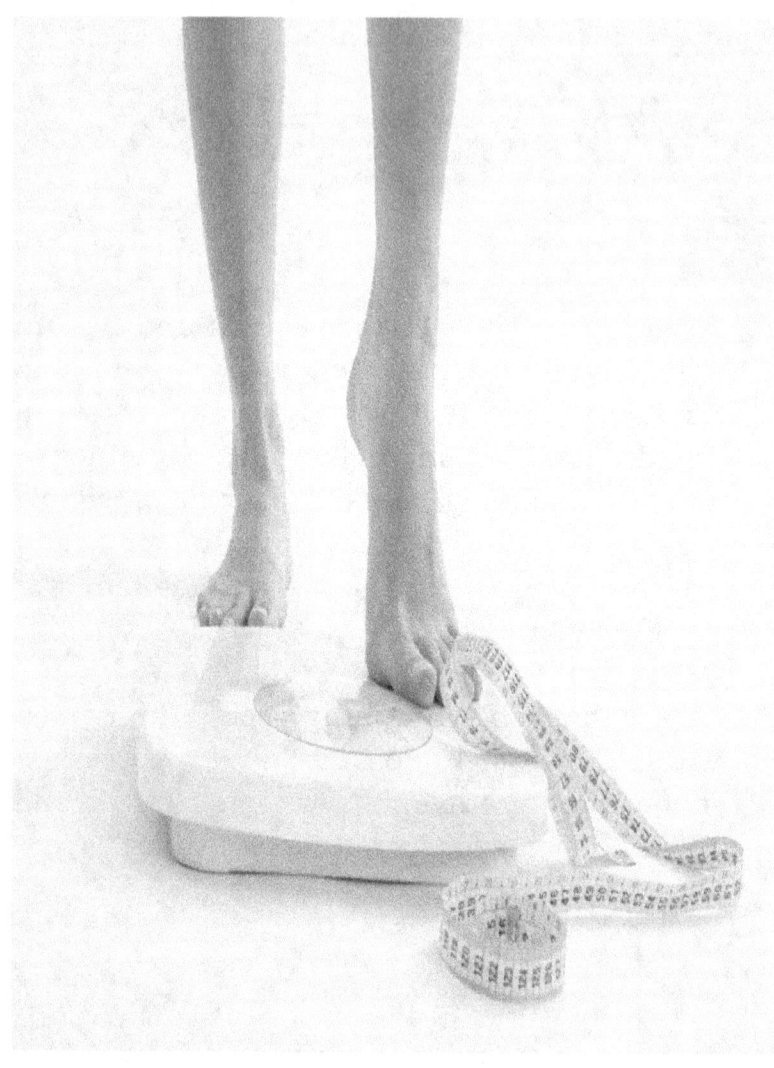